I0436451

The In's and Out's of Coconut Oil:

A Beginners Guide

To Exploring the Amazing Benefits of
Coconut Oil
Help with Weight Loss, Allergies,
Healthier Skin, Hair and much more

by Simone Donovan
http://simonedonovan.com/

The In's and Out's of Coconut Oil

Copyright © 2013

Other Books From This Author

Modern Paleo Book 1: A Beginners Guide to the Paleo Diet

Modern Paleo Book 2: An Athletic Approach To The Paleo Diet

Start Living Gluten Free: A Beginners Guide to a Gluten Free Diet

Book Bundles:

In's and Out's of Coconut Oil and Modern Paleo Beginner's Guide Book Bundle

Modern Paleo Book Bundle

The In's and Out's of Coconut Oil, Modern Paleo The Beginner's Guide and Athletic Approach Book Bundle

Simone Donovan
http://simonedonovan.com/

Contents

The In's and Out's of Coconut Oil

Introduction

As the world continues to evolve technologically, it also grows scientifically. Each day a new study unfolds regarding what is good for your body, and what you should stop using altogether.

Although it is sometimes hard to traverse the statistical studies and understand what is right and what is wrong, there are a few age old secrets that make their way into the lives of the latest generations.

While previous generations swear by their lifelong secret, others have never heard of the benefits of coconut oil. It is fair to say that although it has been used for thousands of years, coconut oil - like most oils, foods and products available everywhere - have fallen in and out of favor with dieticians, physicians and research studies for as long as such professions have existing.

For all the great things coconut oil can bring to your diet and physical appearance, another study will exist countering the claims of its composition. This is not unusual. Everyone cannot agree on everything, and coconut oil isn't any different.

However, it is an all-natural emollient that has been used faithfully by generations of island cultures throughout the world. It is time that coconut oil received its due, and this book aims to provide this exceptional, easy to use oil with its proper representation. Let's dive right in.

Chapter One

Coconut Oil

What is Coconut Oil?

Coconut oil is an edible oil that is extracted from the "meat" of the coconut once it has matured and been harvested from the coconut palm. This delicious and natural extract contains anti-aging benefits, as well as moisturizing and lubricating advantages to anyone who has access to it.

Luckily, it is available in stores and online, so shimmying up a coconut palm is no longer a prerequisite for enjoying its attributes.

Coconuts palms exist in tropical regions, and have been harvested for centuries for their palm leaves that are used as protection from the sun. These palms are sturdy and manipulative, which means they can bend and fold in a number of shapes to form hats, shelter and baskets for transporting goods.

The palm's delicious and nutritious coconuts can be eaten, used as moisturizer, as medicine and for industrial purposes, depending on how they are processed.

History of Coconut Oil

Coconut oil has been used for cooking, pharmaceuticals, and beauty products for approximately 4000 years. The coconut itself has long been harvested for its fruity and delicious flesh while the water and milk within the shell served as a sweet hydration option.

The oil that is derived from the all-purpose coconut has been used for cooking, medical purposes and as a moisturizer in South and Central America, the Caribbean, Polynesia and most of Asia since it was discovered nearly 4000 years ago.

In fact, Europeans believed that it was the coconut oil that delivered the beauty in the people of these geographical areas because their skin, hair and complexion was always so beautiful – and it was the one topical and ingestible agent they all had in common. Later these areas learned to harvest the oil and sell it to the United States and other countries that did not benefit from it being a natural resource.

Coconut oil began descending as a healthy food alternative in the United States in the mid-50s, because of its saturated fat content and the community's shunning of the supposedly hazardous fat altogether.

Saturated fat has become a four letter word in today's society, as misinformed individuals simply believe any labeling of the sort is a poor addition to their diet. What they do not know is that not all saturated fat is a "bad" fat, and that the body needs it to work optimally.

Coconut oil supplies these "good" saturated fats for individuals to ingest safely, so the benefits are received effortlessly.

With the facts revealed, as they will be throughout this book, coconut oil has once again elevated to the top of menus everywhere, and has cemented its place as a healthy alternative to other oils on the market.

What's more is that coconut oil has revealed itself as an exciting beauty aid, providing the beauty secrets of Polynesian princesses to those who have never even seen a coconut palm.

It is an exciting addition to any pantry or medicine cabinet throughout the world, and can literally become a substitute for most topical treatments and beauty components in any home.

Types of Coconut Oil

With its emergence into the limelight once again, coconut oil is providing numerous benefits to its users in the form of nutrition and beauty. Depending on how you plan to use it, you can choose from two different types: Refined and Unrefined.

Refined Coconut Oil

Refined coconut oil is derived from the coconut itself through a process called RBD: Refined, Bleached and Deodorized.

The oil is obtained from the dried coconut flesh, also called "copra". The copra is placed in a press, and heat is added to release the oil.

As it processes, the flavor and the scent are erased as well. The crude oil that is delivered from the copra isn't suitable for consumption, and must be processed again with additional heating and filtering to remove contaminates that arise during the initial drying period.

To obtain the most oil, some brands use chemical solvents to extract as much oil as possible from the meat. RBD oil is used for home cooking, commercial food processing, and cosmetic, industrial, and pharmaceutical purposes.

Unrefined Coconut Oil

Unrefined coconut oil is often referred to as "virgin" or "pure" coconut oil. It is coconut oil extracted from fresh coconut meat rather than its dried counterpart, and is considered a "wet" process.

The fresh coconut meat undergoes one of two processes: wet milling or quick drying. Quick drying, the most common method used, promptly dries the coconut meat and the oil is mechanically expressed in its virgin form, instead of using chemicals to get the most from its natural form.

Wet milling refers to the process in which the coconut milk is expressed from the fresh meat and then boiled, fermented or separated from the milk using enzymes or centrifuge.

Due to the quick process, the resulting oil does not require bleaching or additives. It also isn't exposed to high heat levels like its unrefined counterpart. It retains the distinct flavor and odor of coconut.

When companies produce coconut oil for industrial purposes, the "dry" extraction is typically the preferred method, as it nets approximately 15% more product than the "wet" extraction process.

However, if you are using coconut oil in the

home for consumption or personal beauty applications, the virgin, unrefined option is the best solution available to insure you are receiving each of the benefits the coconut oil has to offer.

Chapter Two

Digestion and Healing

Dietary Benefits

The dietary and health benefits of coconut oil are numerous and exciting, especially for those who suffer from digestive issues including irritable bowel syndrome and chronic indigestion.

In addition, it can help boost the overall immune system to help its users lead a healthier life by fighting infections internally before they can become an outward issue.

Digestive Assistance

Coconut oil is absorbed internally when it is used in foods, or simply ingested whole with a spoon. The latter process is completely safe, and can be consumed daily straight from it packaging, if adding it to foods isn't an option.

This is sometimes the case when you are feeding

an entire family, as other members of your home may scoff at the idea of using coconut oil instead of butter on their toast. There are a number of ways to add the exciting oil to your diet, so adapting the benefits to your diet are easier than you think.

When it is consumed, it helps line the digestive tract to prevent stomach and intestinal problems, including irritable bowel syndrome. In addition, the saturated fats that exist within the oil contain anti-microbial properties that help scour the digestive system of bacteria, parasites and fungi that can cause indigestion and an upset stomach.

Finally, the saturated fats help the body absorb additional amino acids, vitamins and nutrients each time it is consumed. Simply put, you are receiving the benefits of the vitamins and minerals you consume through vegetables, fruits and proteins in their entirety each time you eat when coconut oil is a part of your diet.

Boosts the Immune System

A healthy immune system can make all of the difference in whether you fall victim to illnesses or infections that are caused by outside sources.

Whether it is a seasonal cold, or a lingering infection within the body, coconut oil will help eradicate the body's ability to helplessly succumb to either sidelining event. Coconut oil contains anti-microbial lipids, lauric acid, capric acid and caprylic acid which have anti-fungal, antibacterial and antiviral properties.

The human body converts lauric acid into monolaurin which is claimed to help in dealing with viruses and bacteria causing diseases such as herpes, influenza, and even HIV.

It also helps fight bacteria from the inside of your digestive system, so they are unable to manifest into an infection or illness elsewhere in the body. A healthy immune system is important in fighting any type of infection from the inside out.

Keeping your core healthy will assist in better sleeping habits and reduced anxiety while helping with digestive regularity, so you are free to move about your city or one you are visiting each day without worrying about finding a bathroom.

When your immune system is healthy, you are able to spend more time enjoying life, and less time suffering from colds, infections or even allergies. This natural solution can help deliver you from ailments that have followed you throughout life and help you reclaim your independence naturally.

Healing Properties

Coconut oil isn't only used in the kitchen, it is used topically to help heal damaged tissue, bruising and cuts. When applied directly to the injured area, coconut oil delivers a protective layer that keeps dust, bacteria and fungi from penetrating the wound.

As it protects, it speeds up the healing process. What's more is that its natural anti-fungal and antibiotic properties actually heal the injured area, in addition to providing a second, protective "skin".

Fights Infection

The anti-fungal, antiviral and antibacterial properties of coconut oil make it a great tool in fighting infection. Coconut oil kills the viruses that cause the flu, measles and hepatitis, while delivering a bacteria killing element that heals sore throats, ulcers, urinary tract infections and pneumonia.

Simply adding a teaspoon to your tea can help reduce swelling in the throat, while providing a soothing coat to assist in swallowing. That coating follows the digestive tract, providing a comforting and healing glaze over an existing ulcer, while preventing a new one from arising.

It exits the body through waste, and when it does so, it serves as an elixir to the urinary tract and colon to insure its healing properties are apparent throughout the body.

When used topically, the anti-fungal element of coconut oil can rid athlete's foot and diaper rash quickly and effectively, without irritating the skin.

It is also a great topical remedy for yeast infections, poison ivy and chicken pox, as it soothes the itch of each while providing a natural ointment that heals and protects the infected areas.

Chapter Three

Cholesterol

Practical Approach to Cholesterol

Maintaining a healthy cholesterol level is a key component to one's overall health. Physicians and health enthusiasts alike agree that cholesterol is a dangerous indicator of poor health, and can lead to serious medical issues going forward including strokes, heart attacks and diabetes.

The essential tool in maintaining a healthy cholesterol level is knowing which fats are "good" and which ones are not, so you are ingesting a balanced diet to aid in the existence of proper cholesterol levels.

Promoting Healthy Cholesterol Levels

As most of the western world shied away from using coconut oil because of its high saturated fat count, they forgot to look a little deeper into exactly what those fats delivered. In the case of coconut oil it meant a high level - nearly 50% of its total composition - of lauric acid.

Lauric acid is a type of saturated fat - or fatty acid - that aids in the healing of viral infections, influenza, common colds, fever blisters, cold sores, genital herpes, bronchitis, yeast infections, chlamydia, gonorrhea, and intestinal infections.

With over half of the coconut oil's composition existing as lauric acid, how could one ever go wrong with its use?

The truth about coconut oil is that its natural properties help fight infections from the inside of the body, which means they hardly have time to manifest into a full-blown disruption to your health when used regularly.

As with most true remedies, taking a proactive approach in its use greatly diminishes the risk of infections taking hold to begin with.

Simply put, ingesting coconut oil regularly is the equivalent of applying sunscreen before you get burned, or adding gasoline to your car before it runs out.

The idea of adding coconut oil to your diet is to supply the body with the nutrients and fatty acids it needs to operate optimally, instead of waiting for your cholesterol or blood pressure to spike to dangerous levels before adopting a remedy. The best part is, it is a completely natural elixir, which means there are no side effects or costly expenses incurred with its use.

The Importance of "Good" Fats

Just like every other organ, there is a delicate

balance of good and bad intake throughout the body. The digestive system needs its share of "good" bacteria in order to operate functionally, and the heart needs "good" fats to insure that it performs optimally.

The good fat that is found in coconut oil increases the HDL cholesterol – also known as the "good" cholesterol – in the blood to improve the overall cholesterol ratio levels so the bad never outweighs the good.

In addition, good fats help line the arteries to help reduce injury to the fragile blood lines to deliver decreased occurrences of atherosclerosis, or blockages that can cause clots, strokes and heart attacks.

Coconut oil not only provides the good fats that help the organs work at a maximum level, but it also serves as a lubricant throughout the arteries. The oil, even when ingested in small amounts each day, coats the internal artery walls to keep the blood pumping smoothly, so clots and blockages become a thing of the past. When you are not worried about these two possibly deadly occurrences, you can enjoy life with a fresh approach and a new attitude towards wellness.

Chapter Four

Let's Talk About "Fats"

The Missing Element in Today's Diet?

If there is a single word that any health enthusiast or practical dieter is terrified of, it is the word "fat".

The problem is, not all fats are bad, including saturated fats like those that exist so heavily in coconut oil. It is important to say that keeping an eye on your fat intake is important.

As part of a healthy diet, most individuals are allotted sixty grams of fat per day, and staying within that range can help maintain a healthy weight going forward. When it comes to adding saturated fats to your diet, it is important to do so intelligently and coconut oil is probably the smartest version available.

Saturated Fats: Facts & Misinformation

If the mere mention of saturated fat has you running for the hills, you are misinformed about its necessity in everyone's diet. If this is the case, do not beat yourself up about not knowing better.

The media, dieting guidelines and other misinformed people spread the stigma of saturated fats throughout the community, so it is hard to know what good fat is and what is bad.

The truth is that cutting saturated fat – say swapping bacon for a bagel at breakfast – only increases the triglyceride levels and carbohydrates consumed by the practitioner. In turn, this leads to a decrease in the good, HDL cholesterol.

The body needs the right kind of fats to obtain a balanced approach to internal health, and saturated fats fit into that category beautifully when consumed properly. This means it is more about what you eat than it is about the actual consumption of saturated fats.

If you eat an egg and piece of bacon for breakfast, you are personally balancing your good saturated fat and your omega-3s naturally.

However, if you eat eight strips of bacon on toast, with a tablespoon of mayonnaise slathered between the two, you are ingesting more than your share of saturated fat – and none of it is good.

Likewise, if you are eating fast food every day, you are getting the wrong kinds of saturated fat, and none of it is providing the benefits your body deserves from the "good" versions that are available to everyone.

However, if you swap vegetable oil for coconut

oil, you are introducing a highly concentrated and beneficial saturated fat to your diet.

The overall problem with lumping saturated fats together is exactly that - lumping. It is fair to say that the world has learned that lumping types of people, products, foods and vitamins into categories creates a dangerous generalization.

When it comes to saturated fats, there are too many in existence to make the generalization that all are bad for you. Some really do have exciting and rewarding benefits.

Mono-unsaturated Fatty Acids

In the world of good fats and bad fats, mono-unsaturated fatty acids or MUFAs are a great fat. These fats are derived from the delicious and perfectly healthy staples of avocados, nuts, and olive oil and, of course, coconut oil.

The benefits of MUFAs include:
- Decreased Joint Pain & Stiffness
- Decreased Risk of Breast Cancer
- Improved Circulation
- Lowered Cholesterol Levels
- Lowered Risk for Heart Disease & Stroke
- Reduced Belly Fat
- Weight Loss

All signs point to great things when mono-unsaturated fatty acids are introduced to a healthy diet, especially when they can be derived naturally.

Poly-unsaturated Fatty Acids

Mostly found in sunflower, corn oils and as a substantive segment of the omega-3s in walnuts and salmon, poly-unsaturated fatty acids, or PUFAs, have been shown to lower cholesterol and the overall risk of heart disease by lower triglyceride levels. PUFAs also help build cell membranes to case the arteries and diminish the opportunity for blood clots and inflammation.

Chapter Five

Healthy Applications

The Health of Coconut Oil

When you talk about your overall health it is important to consider your mind, bones and weight as part of its constitution. You may not be at risk for heart disease, but that certainly does not mean that you are not a candidate for osteoporosis later in life.

Your complete health is important to your livelihood and your well-being, which is why the addition of coconut oil can be so beneficial to the masses.

Its health and beauty application provides a boost to the immune system and makes your hair shinier, but what else can it do? More than you could ever imagine.

Weight Loss

It may not be a magic dose of oil, but coconut oil certainly has a number of weight loss benefits that can be extracted from its use. Coconut oil is comprised of short and medium chain fatty acids, which helps remove excessive weight.

In addition, it eases the digestive system so foods − and their vitamins and nutrients − are absorbed easily while boosting enzymes and thyroid functionality. This means you will get the most of what you eat throughout the day, as the body's ability to absorb the nutrients that fruits and vegetable provides will be delivered exactly where they are needed throughout your body.

Meanwhile, another bonus for weight loss enthusiasts is that it delivers less stress to the pancreas, so coconut oil literally increases the metabolism. This allows those who consume it to burn more calories as a result thanks to their increased energy expenditures.

Coconut oil will not make you thinner the moment you begin using it, but it will help kick start your metabolism and help you stay energized longer. This is perfect for pre-workout meals, especially if you are participating in a lengthy physical event including a race on foot, bike or in the water.

Depression

Depression can be caused by a number of sources, and when weight, stiffness and immobility are factors, coconut oil can help diffuse their involvement. As it helps boost your metabolism, weight loss becomes a genuine side effect of its use. This allows you to feel better, look better and improve your overall self-esteem to help battle previously depressive areas of life.

In addition, as it counters thyroid issues – which have a side effect of depression - coconut oil is able to diminish two physical issues at once, allowing for a healthier life to emerge on the other side of its intake. The soothing application of coconut oil, and its overall ingestion, also helps reduce anxiety which can play a large role in depression.

Osteoporosis

The consumption of coconut oil drastically increases the body's ability to absorb key vitamins and nutrients including calcium and magnesium which help develop stronger bones, and ward off the risk of osteoporosis. It also helps reduce joint pain so you are able to stay physically active and ward off any bone decomposition that may result from a sedentary lifestyle.

Taking a cue from the old expression, "Use it or lose it" coconut oil helps keep you active, without the accompanying pain you may have felt before when practicing the same activities.

Heart Health

Thanks to the aforementioned lauric acid composition of coconut oil, not only does it coat the arteries to avoid injury and help balance the "good" cholesterol, but it also helps alleviate the propensity for high blood pressure that can cause heart disease and strokes.

Since coconut oil contains fewer calories than other oils it dissolves easily thereby forgoing the accumulation of fat in the arteries. This means fewer chances of blockages, and a smoother flow of blood to and from the heart and the balance of the circulatory systems.

When blood is flowing throughout the body at an optimal level, it prevents cramping and aching, which means you are able to become more active throughout the day. It also helps provide a sound sleeping arrangement, as leg cramps and sore joints are two usual suspects when it comes to sleepless nights. Getting rid of both will help you rest easier and more soundly each time you go to bed.

Alzheimer's Disease & Dementia

Alzheimer's disease and dementia have been regarded as diabetic conditions in the brain. Insulin and glucose are two major factors in the diseases' progression, and the fact that there isn't cure for any of the three afflictions help them draw parallel descriptions.

The amount of insulin produced by a patient who suffers from either one of these diseases blocks the glucose from reaching the brain, which causes the cells to degrade and eventually die. This degradation contributes to memory loss and confusion. The ketones in coconut oil are metabolized in the liver, and expanded to the brain to allow for the acceptance of glucose.

This process thereby enlivens the sensors and cells to help them operate actively and avoid degradation. This process and the resulting "moving mind" helps nurture the memory and overall well-being of the brain, allowing Alzheimer's and dementia to be warded off for extended periods.

Since the symptoms of these diseases typically do not evolve into well after the damage is done, it is important to provide the brain with a proper defense, and coconut oil does exactly that

Diabetes

Coconut oil helps control blood sugar levels, which means it improves the natural secretion of insulin. It also effectively utilizes blood glucose which helps prevent and treat diabetic conditions naturally.

For those who are not diabetic, but simply get light headed or even grouchy when they have missed a meal, coconut oil can help keep you fuller, longer, so those stubborn side effects do not come into play as often.

It also keeps you from making snap decisions on snacking, which typically leads to quick and unhealthy options when you are on the go.

Organ Care: Liver and Kidneys

Thanks to the medium chain triglycerides and fatty acids that comprise coconut oil, it can help deliver organ care throughout the body. First, it is easily converted to energy which keeps the liver from working so hard to break down the bad fats, thereby preventing the accumulation of fat around the liver and subsequently lowering the risk of liver diseases.

Next, the kidneys benefits from its consumption by dissolving kidney stones and hardened accumulations helping to prevent kidney and gallbladder diseases.

Other internal assistance attributed to coconut oil is:

- Bladder Health

- Improves Sperm Motility & Fertility
- Prostate Health
- Protect Against Cancer
- Protect Against Food Poisoning
- Protect Against Seizures
- Protect Against Toxic Shock Syndrome
- Reduce Inflammation
- Reduce Sinus Infections

Internal care isn't the only reason, although it is a great one, to consider adding coconut oil to your diet. It can also benefit the outer you in the form of a beauty aid for the hair, skin and teeth.

Chapter Six

Beauty Applications

The Beauty of Coconut Oil

The benefits of coconut oil are seemingly endless, especially when it comes maintaining your outer beauty. One of the first things people consider when dealing with beauty maintenance is their hair.

Women and men alike spend an exorbitant amount of time insuring their hair is straight or curly, smooth and shiny and basically in the best shape possible to draw the attention of passersby.

Everyone loves a great mane of hair, and that isn't lost on a single individual in today's world. The good news is, everyone can have it with the help of coconut oil.

Applying coconut oil to wet hair as a conditioner helps the overall health of the hair, and provides a shiny outcome once it dries. It not only helps maintain healthy hair, but helps re-grow damaged hair to a healthier state by reducing the loss of protein that most hair care products will strip away unknowingly.

What's more is that it adds significant amounts of the essential proteins that are necessary to reverse the signs of damage. With each addition use, coconut oil protects the hair from the elements, blow drying and hot irons that are popular in most vanities around the world.

As a natural form of SPF, it can also assist with protecting the hair from damaging UV rays that could spoil a fresh coloring or the hair's overall health.

Coconut oil is also great for taming frizz, flyaway strands and static once the hair is already dry. Simply place a tiny amount in between your fingers and rub your hands together, as you would with a store bought pomade, and dab the problem areas accordingly.

It also adds a lovely scent to your final 'do and delivers a soft appearance so the existence of "product" isn't apparent or unsightly.

These essential oils and proteins work even harder at repairing dry and damaged scalps that produce dandruff as a result of their arid composition. When coconut oil is applied topically and massage directly into the scalp it helps prevent dandruff and dry scalp from reoccurring.

The best part is it will also keep the scalp clean from head lice and their eggs by effectively killing any existing lice and preventing their return with continued use.

Coconut Oil & Skin Care

If you, like most individuals, are looking to ward off the signs of aging including dryness, wrinkles, age spots, discoloration and sagging skin, look no further than coconut oil to help you look younger, faster.

It has been said, depending on your skin type, that a mere spoonful of coconut oil can moisturize the entire body. Certainly the results will vary for everyone, as will the amounts that you use, but try applying it minimally at first to see what works for you on different parts of the body.

You certainly cannot use too much, as it absorbs into the skin quickly because it is an all-natural emollient.

Moisturizer

Apply coconut oil to your face to diminish wrinkles, sun spots and discoloration. You can tap the solution under your eyes to remove "bags" or dark circles beginning with the first application.

Apply it to your elbows and hands to remove signs of aging and dryness that typically affect those two areas more than most. It also helps diminish the appearance of darkening skin around the knees and elbows that increases with age.

Applying coconut oil to your hands will improve nail growth and strength, while massaging the cuticles to enliven the nail beds. When applied to feet it can repair even the roughest heels, while ridding the toes and bottoms of athlete's foot or fungi related problems quickly, effectively and naturally.

Coconut oil is also great for sunburns, as its effective moisturizing composition will help deliver relief with a single application. It is also a natural SPF 4, so can be used before going for a walk to help your skin repel the sun before it has the opportunity to burn.

Acne & Skin Conditions

The natural antioxidants that are available in coconut oil can do more than soften the skin and help reduce the signs of aging. It can also help treat acne, eczema, psoriasis, dermatitis and skin infections that may have previously hindered your confidence.

Simply apply it topically to the areas of concern, and allow the natural remedy to do the rest. The anti-microbial composition of coconut oil allows it to act as a natural anti-oxidant and anti-biotic. That means that it not only soothes the dryness upon contact, but it actually helps heal the irritated skin at the source, you can start feeling and looking better in no time. Use it on your face, arms, and chest and wherever skin is irritated to help the healing process begin.

Stretch Marks & Varicose Veins

If there is one solution that has been passed down from generation to generation it is that coconut oil helps prevent stretch marks before they can become an issue, and effectively lightens any that have already made their way onto the skin.

As with any serum, using it preventively will help your chances of avoiding whatever affliction you are aiming to disguise in the first place. In this case, it is stretch marks.

Stretch marks can be the result of muscle gain, weight gain, weight loss and the overall evolution of the body. As you age, the body begins to change rapidly in different areas than you remember, and stretch marks can appear as a result before you even know it.

Coconut oil can help treat stretch marks by simply applying it to the source of the markings. No matter when the stretch marks are, it is safe to apply coconut oil, as it does not disrupt the body's flora as a result of its use.

If it is pregnancy that has you worried about obtaining stretch marks, simply rub the coconut oil onto your belly during gestation, and continue to apply it as the months go along to avoid stretch marks altogether.

If you were not able to read this before the adaptation of stretch marks, it certainly isn't too late to get rid of them. Simply rub coconut oil on the affected areas and watch in delight as your stretch marks begin to lighten, and eventually disappear altogether.

Coconut oil not only suppresses the appearance of stretch marks, but it can also reduce the signs of varicose veins by lighting the appearance of dark veins on the surface of the skin. It is also been shown to help reduce the signs of cellulite on the legs, buttocks and hips.

Simply apply coconut oil as you would a regular moisturizer, and allow it to work its magic. The worst that can happen is that your skin will be incredibly moisturized as a result of its use.

Safe for Babies

If you are pregnant and planning to breastfeed after the baby is born, it will not take long to realize that the breasts and nipples will become dry and irritated as a result.

Coconut oil is a perfect moisturizer for such a tender area of the body, and it is completely safe for your child, so you do not have to worry about any adverse reactions during or after feedings.

Simply coat the nipple after feedings to help moisturize before the baby's next meal.

Once the child is here, coconut oil can also be used directly on the baby's bottom when diaper rash occurs, as it provides a natural healing process to the affected area with the very first use.

Much like adults can use coconut oil on their heads to suppress dandruff and moisturize the scalp, babies can benefit from the same application to prevent or heal cradle cap naturally. It can also be applied to dry areas of their tiny, sensitive bodies without the worry of irritation.

Shaving

Since coconut oil is considered a lubricant in some capacities, it makes for perfect shaving oil for anywhere you would like to apply a razor.

Simply apply the coconut oil to the skin, and shave over the area with a clean razor to receive a close, long lasting shave.

Removal of Make Up

For some, removing make up can be a hazardous instance of rubbing too hard or using harsh astringents to insure that there aren't any lingering patches of color left behind. Coconut oil can help lubricate the skin, much like it does when shaving.

The lubricating properties allow you to apply it to your face with your fingers or a cotton applicator, and wiping away even the deepest mascara applications in one swipe. This proven approach to make up removal is even used on stage performers to insure that all of the heavy applications are left backstage, while leaving the skin smooth without the fear of irritation.

Lubricant

Since coconut oil is a perfect lubricant for removing make up, it is also a perfect actual lubricant for massages or sex.

It is a natural, sensual moisturizer that is safe to use on all areas of the body, so you do not have to take care in where it is applied. It also has a nice scent, so massages become an aromatherapy dream.

Finally, coconut oil can be used as a natural alternative to Chap Stick, and will leave your lips soft, supple and healthy as a result of repeated use.

Teeth

It may sound silly to apply any oils to your teeth, in any form, but many eastern cultures have been doing it for thousands of years to help maintain dental health.

The process is called "oil pulling" and is completed by adding approximately one tablespoon of coconut oil to the mouth and swishing it around the teeth and gums for ten minutes or so.

In effect, the oil catches the bacteria and dissolves it with its anti-microbial composition, which kills bacteria, fungi and viruses including gingivitis and plaque.

The consistent use of coconut oil pulling has been determined to stifle tooth decay as well, which means fewer trips to the dentist.

Finally, since coconut oil provides better vitamin and nutrient consumption within the body, you will be getting more calcium, which helps strengthen teeth.

Chapter Seven

Coconut Oil and Cooking

The Benefits of Coconut Oil & Dieting

If you are on a diet, are an athlete or body builder, coconut oil should be your go-to fuel before and after workouts. Even if you are a Paleo dieter, coconut oil is an approved addition to your meals, and should be enjoyed through cooking all of your favorite veggies and lean meats, while adding a tasty approach to dining.

Dieters can enjoy the fact that coconut oil contains fewer calories than other oils, and since its fatty acids are consumed quickly and converted to energy instead of accumulated fat, it basically serves as fuel.

Coconut oil also helps boost energy levels and enhances endurance and performance in athletes so long distance runners and weight lifters can enjoy the same benefits in differing capacities.

Cooking with Coconut Oil

One of the best reasons to cook with coconut oil, besides its immense health benefits, is that it is incredibly stable and can last for months without going bad. This means you can invest in a large quantity, using it throughout the entire home, without worrying about waste.

You can also use it to cook at high temperatures, without worrying about the smoke point becoming overwhelming, and it tastes really good! The same cannot be said for olive oil, as it typically burns quicker than coconut oil and can char your foods as a result.

It can be used for baking, sautéing and pan-searing foods effortlessly, while providing the essential benefits of the good saturated fats your body will appreciate.

To cook with coconut oil, you will simply use it in the place of butter, vegetable or canola oils, grease and especially lard. As a standard note to anyone who would like to keep their arteries unclogged, you should never use lard.

Coconut oil can be added to a pan just as you would olive oil when you are ready to sauté vegetables and fruits. It can also be melted and added to vegetables that are being roasted on the grille or in the oven.

Simply melt the oil in a pan or microwave, toss the vegetables and place them on the grille in aluminum foil or in an oven safe pan for roasting beautifully delicious and nutritious side dishes.

Both of these practices can be applied to fish and lean meats when they are being prepared for meals as well.

Simply drizzle the oil into a skillet to sear meats and fish. Add it to the outside of chicken as a rub to provide a great tenderness when roasting in the oven or on the grill.

When you would like to use coconut oil instead of butter or margarine – as requested in most baked goods' recipes – simply melt one cup of coconut oil for every one liquid cup needed for the baking recipe.

The added benefit – besides the numerous ones to your health – of using the oil in baked goods is that it enhances the moisture level ten-fold, which is perfect for cakes, brownies, pies and cookies. It also delivers a tasty flavor of the tropics that is subtle, so it does not overwhelm anyone who does not like coconut.

Another exciting use for coconut oil in the kitchen is lining baking pans and seasoning cast iron pans and skillets. This perfectly natural oil will help provide a clean release for all sorts of dessert treats from muffins to macaroons without leaving a greasy feel to the pan or the treats.

Benefits over the "Other Oils"

Other oils and even butter will supply your meals with moisture so they cook without burning, but none of the other oils will provide the health benefits of coconut oil.

Vegetable oil and margarine are simply not good for you. In fact, most are genetically modified and include preservatives, fats and sodium that are no more natural than the package they are sold in.

Vegetable oils are also a contributing factor in disturbing the omega-6 and omega-3 ratio. When there is an overabundance of the omega-6 in a person's diet, they can suffer from heart disease, high blood pressure and artery damage. There are no real health benefits derived from consuming either, so simply skip the meaningless step in the kitchen and turn to coconut oil as a health substitute.

Olive oil and flax seed oil are approved Paleo Diet additions, and have some nutritional value in the form of mono-unsaturated fats.

However, so does coconut oil. The latter also provides more health benefits and a tasty flavor to any of your culinary creations and helps keep your overall saturated fats in check with each use. In with the good fats, and out with the bad.

Cooking Temperature Comparisons

One of the great things about cooking with coconut oil is that it has a standard smoke point to that of olive oil, which means it can withstand a hot oven without setting off the smoke detector!

Actually, when oils get hot, they begin to break down which means they are losing their nutritional value as the temperature rises.

Not to worry, however. Unrefined coconut oil has a smoke point as high as 350 degrees and its refined counterpart as high as 450 degrees.

Here is how that compares to other cooking oil options:

Vegetable Shortening (Hydrogenated)	325°F
Butter	350°F
Lard	375°F
Olive Oil	325°F - 375°F
Corn Oil	400°F - 450°F
Canola Oil	425°F - 475°F
Clarified Butter	450°F - 475°F
Sunflower Oil	450°F - 475°F
Soybean Oil	450°F - 475°F
Safflower Oil	475°F - 500°F

This allows you to cook with coconut oil effortlessly, without making a mess of your meal, or your kitchen.

It also allows you to add flavor to average foods like kale and fish, providing a gourmet finishing touch to your dieting and sprucing up even the most bland cuisine options with very little effort.

Coconut Oil & Your Workout

In addition to providing an endurance and energy boost, coconut oil allows each of your organs to operate optimally so you get the most out of your workouts. The best approach to adding coconut oil to your diet to help your workout and weight loss potential is drizzling it over your morning oatmeal (or meal preference of your choice) to jump start your metabolism.

It will also help suppress hunger, so you can get to your next meal without splurging on fatty quick fix snacks in between.

Before you work out, add coconut oil to your diet to increase your energy and enhance your endurance, so you can burn through calories more efficiently than you would without it.

This is a perfectly safe way to add energy-based fats to your diet without consuming carbs so your body can work out optimally. It will allow you to power through your workout, without feeling overwhelmed or exhausted. Consume it by the spoonful or in a smoothie to get your workout underway with a blast of positive energy.

After your workout, add coconut oil to your protein shake to add healthy, mass building fats to your diet effectively. It will help repair tired muscles, and keep injury at bay so your tired body has time to heal before you hit the gym again.

If you are feeling really banged up from your workout, add a tablespoon of coconut oil to a hot bath to help you relax and cure the external pain naturally. If you are growing mass quickly, and your body is showing growth in muscular areas, rub coconut oil directly on the growing segments to reduce stretch marks.

Fun Ways to Add Coconut Oil to Your Diet & Kitchen

When you are not using coconut oil to sauté vegetables or to grease pans for baking or pan-searing fish, there are a number of ways to substitute your usual butter, oil or moisture application with beneficial and delicious coconut oil.

- Fry, Scramble or Omelets and Egg
- Grilled Cheese Sandwiches
- Popcorn Topping

- Spread it on Toast & Muffins
- Sweeten Coffee or Tea
- Top Salads
- Season and Moisturize Wooden Cutting Boards
- Top Fruits like Berries and Melons
- Add to Stir Fry Entrees
- Use with Pancakes & Waffles

Consider using coconut oil each time you reach for olive oil or butter to add to a meal. The health benefits are numerous, and the taste is amazing!

There are also a number of opportunities to use coconut oil outside of your diet, including:

- Clean BBQ Grilles
- Furniture Polish
- Gum Removal (from hair, furniture, rugs and carpet)
- Insect Repellent
- Leather Moisturizer
- Lubricate (similar to WD-40) Zippers, Bike Chains & Stubborn Sticking Points
- Metal Polish
- Polish Shoes
- Prevent Freezer Burn
- Remove Wax, Sap and Sticky Items
- Stain Removal (Goo Gone Alternative)

The exciting benefits of coconut oil aren't simply for you. If you have a pet, he or she can benefit from its consumption as well. Coconut oil delivers all of the benefits to pets that it does humans, which means your furry friend can receive a boost of energy for long walks or hikes.

In addition, it delivers a shiny coat and reduces hairball potential in cats. It also delivers fresh breath to man's best friend, without using alcohol based sprays or harmful ingredients.

Coconut oil is a great alternative to traditional oils, and can be used in the kitchen, in the bathroom and even in the bedroom, so it will never go to waste around the house.

Some even use the all-purpose oil in the garage to lubricate small parts and machine components to help them run smoothly. You can rub it on door hinges to reduce noisy openings and closings, without suffocating your family with the seemingly toxic smell WD-40 invites, while getting the same results.

With all of the great uses that coconut oil provides, the best part is that it isn't going to hurt you, so you can experiment with it anywhere and everywhere in the home. Add it to your smoothies or rub it in your hair. Moisturize your rough elbows and ankles, and drop a teaspoon onto your morning meal.

There is absolutely no wrong way to use coconut oil, so enjoy its benefits and its incredible taste as often as possible in a myriad versatile ways.

There is literally no wrong way to use coconut oil, so grab a vat of it from your local retailer or favorite online store and start using it everywhere! The less you have to worry about your kids inhaling fumes, or eating something they should not, the better off you will be mentally.

Coconut oil is non-toxic, and allows you to use it on anyone, at any age, to cure the a sore throat or common cold, while boosting their immune system by simply introducing it into their diet.

If you have a picky house, and know that any "new" addition to the kitchen will be met with adversity, use it without telling anyone you have made the switch. Chances are they will not even notice that you are greasing cake pans with something besides cooking spray, or that you are adding it to vegetables before they hit the grille.

Additionally, when your child suffers from a bout of poison ivy, you can revert to the same container and rub the conditioning salve into their infected area to see instant relief.

Coconut oil is a perfect addition to any home, and can be used openly or in disguise, to insure that your family is receiving the benefits they deserve from any store bought household product.

Conclusion

Using coconut oil for a health, beauty and maintenance around your home is a perfectly cost effective solution to the myriad of goods you would buy to cook or treat infections or apply lotions, condition hair and treat acne separately.

One solution for every room in the house seems like a dream come true, and you have nothing to lose by trying it for hundreds of different applications. If it does not work specifically for your condition, it does not mean it will not work for another.

The idea behind coconut oil is that it has worked for generations, and providing amazing results to households around the world. What do you have to lose by picking up a jar of it today?

Worst case, you will be cooking with a sweet and beneficial new oil, and applying it to your hair to insure you are getting a perfectly Polynesian shine each time you leave the house.

The general uses for coconut oil are innumerable, and chances are, you will find your very own uses along the way. Just be sure to share them with family and friends, so everyone can benefit from this inexpensive, all-purpose tonic going forward. You have nothing to lose, and everything to gain from its use, so why not give it a try?

Did You Like This Book?

I hope you learned a few things that will help you in your goals of either losing weight or just to eat healthier from my book.

I would really appreciate it if you would return to the Kindle store and leave a review and rating for this book, because Kindle rankings are driven by readers and customers like you.

I do hope you enjoyed this book and I would love to hear what you thought of it. You can leave your comments here:
http://www.amazon.com/dp/B00E66OLHW

Or you can simply go to Amazon.com and search for "**The In's and Out's of Coconut Oil**", and this book's page will come up.

You May also be interested in other books I have done

Modern Paleo Book 1: A Beginners Guide to the Paleo Diet

Modern Paleo Book 2: An Athletic Approach To The Paleo Diet

Start Living Gluten Free: A Beginners Guide to a Gluten Free Diet

Book Bundles:

In's and Out's of Coconut Oil and Modern Paleo Beginner's Guide Book Bundle

Modern Paleo Book Bundle

The In's and Out's of Coconut Oil, Modern Paleo The Beginner's Guide and Athletic Approach Book Bundle

Thank you so much for purchasing my book.

Simone Donovan
http://simonedonovan.com/